Publisher Information

Copyright © 2025, **DrMed**
All rights reserved.

No part of this book may be reproduced, distributed, or transmitted in any form or by any means, including photocopying, recording, or other electronic or mechanical methods, without the prior written permission of the publisher, except in the case of brief quotations used for review purposes or academic references.

Under no circumstances will any blame or legal responsibility be held against the publisher, or author, for any damages, reparation, or monetary loss due to the information contained within this book, either directly or indirectly.

Before reading the book, please read the disclaimer.

For permissions, inquiries, or other correspondence:
drmedhealth.com@gmail.com

For more information, please visit.
www.DrMedHealth.com

Disclaimer

The content of this book is a work of fiction. Names, characters, places, medical scenarios, and incidents are either the product of the author's imagination or are used fictitiously. Any resemblance to actual persons, living or dead, real-life medical events, organizations, or institutions is purely coincidental.

The medical procedures, treatments, and conditions described are for narrative purposes only and should not be interpreted as professional advice. Readers are advised not to use the medical information presented in this book as a substitute for consulting healthcare professionals or seeking proper medical care.

Neither the author, Dr. Nilesh Panchal, nor the publisher, **DrMedHealth**, assumes any responsibility for actions taken based on the information contained within these novels. Any opinions expressed in the book are solely those of the author and do not represent the views of any affiliated institutions or organizations.

Chapter 1: What are the Most Common Causes of Esophagitis, and How Do They Vary Among Different Age Groups and Populations? 4

Chapter 2: What Symptoms Are Typically Associated with Esophagitis, and How Can They Be Distinguished from Other Gastrointestinal Disorders? 13

Chapter 3: How Does Gastroesophageal Reflux Disease (GERD) Contribute to the Development of Esophagitis, and What Are Its Other Underlying Risk Factors? 23

Chapter 4: What Are the Differences Between the Various Types of Esophagitis, Such as Eosinophilic Esophagitis, Infectious Esophagitis, and Drug-Induced Esophagitis? 33

Chapter 5: What Diagnostic Methods Are Used to Confirm Esophagitis, and How Do Endoscopy, Biopsy, and Imaging Techniques Contribute to Accurate Diagnosis? 43

Chapter 6: How Is Eosinophilic Esophagitis Diagnosed and Treated, and What Role Do Food Allergies and Elimination Diets Play in Its Management? 52

Chapter 8: What Are the Key Treatment Options for Esophagitis, Including Lifestyle Modifications, Medications, and, in Severe Cases, Surgical Interventions? 72

Chapter 9: How Can Esophagitis Be Prevented, and What Steps Can Individuals Take to Minimize Their Risk of Developing This Condition? 84

Chapter 10: Esophagitis: A Comprehensive Clinical Guide for Patients and Practitioners 94

Chapter 1: What are the Most Common Causes of Esophagitis, and How Do They Vary Among Different Age Groups and Populations?

Esophagitis, or inflammation of the esophagus, is a condition that can cause significant discomfort and lead to complications if left untreated. Understanding its causes is essential to effectively manage and prevent the condition. The esophagus serves as a vital conduit, transporting food and liquids from the mouth to the stomach. When it becomes inflamed, swallowing can become painful, and the individual may experience heartburn, chest pain, or regurgitation. This chapter explores the diverse causes of esophagitis, shedding light on how these factors vary across different age groups and populations.

Common Causes of Esophagitis

1. Gastroesophageal Reflux Disease (GERD)

GERD is the most prevalent cause of esophagitis, characterized by the backward flow of stomach acid into the esophagus. This acid reflux irritates the esophageal lining, leading to inflammation. GERD-associated esophagitis is common among adults and is often linked to lifestyle factors such as obesity, smoking, and dietary habits.

- **Mechanism:** The lower esophageal sphincter (LES), a ring of muscle at the junction of the esophagus and stomach, acts as a barrier to prevent acid from traveling upward. When the LES is weakened or relaxes inappropriately, acid reflux occurs, resulting in esophagitis.
- **Risk Factors:** Eating large meals, lying down soon after eating, and consuming fatty or spicy foods are major contributors. Alcohol, caffeine, and certain medications can also relax the LES, exacerbating reflux.

2. Eosinophilic Esophagitis (EoE)

EoE is an allergic condition driven by an overproduction of eosinophils, a type of white blood cell, in the esophageal lining. This form of esophagitis is increasingly recognized in both children and adults.

- **Triggers:** EoE is often linked to food allergies or environmental allergens. Common food triggers include dairy, wheat, eggs, soy, and nuts.
- **Symptoms:** Patients with EoE may experience difficulty swallowing, food impaction, and heartburn that does not respond to typical GERD treatments.
- **Prevalence:** EoE is more common in younger populations, particularly in children and young adults. It is also more frequently diagnosed in males than females.

3. Infectious Esophagitis

Infections can cause esophagitis, especially in individuals with compromised immune systems. The most common infectious agents include:

- **Fungal Infections:** *Candida albicans*, a yeast, is a leading cause of esophagitis in people with weakened immunity, such as those with HIV/AIDS, cancer, or diabetes. It is also seen in individuals on prolonged antibiotic or corticosteroid therapy.
- **Viral Infections:** Viruses such as herpes simplex virus (HSV) and cytomegalovirus (CMV) can infect the esophagus, particularly in immunocompromised individuals.

- **Bacterial Infections:** While less common, bacterial infections can also contribute to esophagitis, often secondary to trauma or other underlying conditions.

4. Drug-Induced Esophagitis

Certain medications can cause esophagitis by irritating the esophageal lining or becoming lodged in the esophagus, causing localized inflammation. This condition is often referred to as "pill-induced esophagitis."

- **Culprit Medications:** Common offenders include nonsteroidal anti-inflammatory drugs (NSAIDs), bisphosphonates (used to treat osteoporosis), tetracycline antibiotics, potassium chloride, and iron supplements.
- **Mechanism:** Improper swallowing technique, such as taking pills without sufficient water or lying down immediately after ingestion, increases the risk.
- **Prevalence:** Drug-induced esophagitis is more common in older adults, who are more likely to take multiple medications.

5. Radiation Esophagitis

Radiation therapy for cancers of the chest, neck, or esophagus can damage the esophageal lining, leading to inflammation. Radiation esophagitis is a common side effect of cancer treatment.

- **Symptoms:** Patients may experience difficulty swallowing, chest pain, and a burning sensation in the esophagus.
- **Duration:** Symptoms often develop during or shortly after radiation therapy and may persist for weeks or months.

6. Chemical Injury

Ingestion of caustic substances, such as household cleaners, acids, or alkalis, can cause severe esophagitis. This is more common in children who accidentally ingest harmful substances or in adults attempting self-harm.

- **Immediate Effects:** Chemical burns can result in severe inflammation, ulceration, and even perforation of the esophagus.
- **Long-Term Risks:** Scarring and strictures may develop, leading to chronic swallowing difficulties.

7. Autoimmune Disorders

Certain autoimmune conditions, such as scleroderma and Crohn's disease, can involve the esophagus and cause esophagitis.

- **Scleroderma:** This condition leads to fibrosis and dysfunction of the esophageal muscles, increasing the risk of reflux and subsequent esophagitis.

- **Crohn's Disease:** Although rare, Crohn's can directly affect the esophagus, causing localized inflammation and ulceration.

Variation by Age Groups

Infants and Children

- **Primary Causes:** Eosinophilic esophagitis and GERD are the leading causes of esophagitis in younger populations. Food allergies play a significant role in pediatric cases of EoE.
- **Symptoms:** Infants may present with feeding difficulties, vomiting, and failure to thrive. Older children might complain of abdominal pain, difficulty swallowing, or regurgitation.
- **Management:** Diagnosis often involves endoscopy and allergy testing. Treatment includes dietary modifications, proton pump inhibitors (PPIs), and topical corticosteroids.

Adults

- **Primary Causes:** GERD is the most common cause of esophagitis in adults. Other contributing factors include

medication use, infections, and autoimmune disorders.
- **Lifestyle Factors:** Obesity, smoking, and alcohol consumption are significant contributors in this age group.
- **Management:** Lifestyle changes, dietary modifications, and medications like PPIs and H2 blockers are common treatments.

Elderly

- **Primary Causes:** Older adults are more prone to drug-induced esophagitis due to polypharmacy and decreased esophageal motility. GERD and infections are also common.
- **Complications:** The elderly are at higher risk for complications such as strictures and Barrett's esophagus.
- **Management:** Careful medication management and monitoring are crucial to prevent pill-induced esophagitis.

Variation by Populations

Geographical Differences

- **Developed Countries:** GERD-related esophagitis is more common due to lifestyle factors like high-fat diets and obesity.
- **Developing Countries:** Infectious esophagitis is more prevalent, often linked

to higher rates of HIV/AIDS and limited access to healthcare.

Ethnic and Genetic Factors

- **Eosinophilic Esophagitis:** Studies suggest that EoE may be more common in individuals of Caucasian descent, potentially due to genetic predisposition and dietary habits.
- **GERD-Related Esophagitis:** Certain populations, such as those of Asian descent, may have a lower prevalence of GERD, possibly due to differences in diet and lifestyle.

Socioeconomic Status

- **Low Socioeconomic Status:** Limited access to healthcare and poor nutrition can increase the risk of infectious and chemical-induced esophagitis.
- **High Socioeconomic Status:** Lifestyle factors like overeating, alcohol consumption, and high-stress levels can contribute to GERD-related esophagitis.

The causes of esophagitis are diverse, ranging from lifestyle-related GERD to immune-mediated conditions like EoE. Age, geographic location, and socioeconomic factors play significant roles in determining the prevalence and type of esophagitis in different populations. By understanding these variations, healthcare providers can develop tailored prevention and treatment strategies to address this common yet complex condition effectively.

Chapter 2: What Symptoms Are Typically Associated with Esophagitis, and How Can They Be Distinguished from Other Gastrointestinal Disorders?

Esophagitis, the inflammation of the esophagus, manifests through a variety of symptoms that can significantly impact an individual's quality of life. Identifying these symptoms accurately is essential for timely diagnosis and effective treatment. This chapter delves into the typical symptoms of esophagitis, their underlying mechanisms, and how they can be differentiated from other gastrointestinal (GI) disorders with overlapping clinical presentations.

Common Symptoms of Esophagitis

1. Dysphagia (Difficulty Swallowing)

Dysphagia is one of the hallmark symptoms of esophagitis. Patients may report a sensation of food "sticking" in their throat or chest during swallowing. This difficulty can range from mild discomfort to severe obstruction, depending on the extent of inflammation and any secondary complications such as strictures or scarring.

- **Mechanism:** Inflammation narrows the esophageal lumen, reducing its ability to accommodate the passage of food and liquids. Severe cases can result in esophageal strictures, further exacerbating the symptom.
- **Differentiation:** Dysphagia in esophagitis is often progressive, worsening with time, whereas in conditions like achalasia or esophageal cancer, it may initially be intermittent or associated with other systemic signs such as weight loss.

2. Odynophagia (Painful Swallowing)

Pain during swallowing, or odynophagia, is another prominent symptom of esophagitis. Patients may describe sharp or burning pain localized to the chest or throat when eating or drinking, particularly with hot, cold, or acidic foods and beverages.

- **Mechanism:** The inflamed esophageal mucosa becomes hypersensitive, and the passage of food or liquids can trigger pain. Ulcers or erosions in the esophagus, common in severe esophagitis, further heighten this discomfort.
- **Differentiation:** Odynophagia in esophagitis is typically provoked by swallowing, unlike the chest pain of cardiac origin, which occurs independently of food intake.

3. Heartburn (Pyrosis)

Heartburn is a burning sensation in the chest that often radiates upward to the throat or neck. It is most commonly associated with GERD-induced esophagitis but can also occur in other forms of the condition.

- **Mechanism:** Acid reflux damages the esophageal lining, causing irritation and the characteristic burning sensation.
- **Differentiation:** Heartburn due to esophagitis tends to occur after meals, particularly large or fatty meals, or when lying down. It is typically relieved by antacids, distinguishing it from cardiac-related chest pain.

4. Regurgitation

Regurgitation, the backflow of food or stomach contents into the mouth or throat, is another common symptom of esophagitis. It is often accompanied by an acidic or bitter taste.

- **Mechanism:** Weakened lower esophageal sphincter (LES) function allows stomach contents to reflux into the esophagus and sometimes reach the throat.
- **Differentiation:** Regurgitation in esophagitis is more likely to involve acidic or bile-stained material, unlike vomiting, which is a forceful expulsion of stomach contents and may indicate other GI disorders like gastroparesis or intestinal obstruction.

5. Chest Pain

Chest pain in esophagitis can mimic cardiac pain, making it a diagnostic challenge. It may be sharp, burning, or pressure-like, located behind the sternum.

- **Mechanism:** Esophageal inflammation irritates local sensory nerves, leading to pain that can radiate to the neck, back, or arms.
- **Differentiation:** Unlike angina, esophageal chest pain is often related to food intake, body position (e.g., lying down), or acid reflux. Relief with antacids is another distinguishing feature.

6. Nausea and Vomiting

While less specific, nausea and vomiting can occur in esophagitis, especially in cases caused by infections or chemical injury.

- **Mechanism:** Severe irritation or ulceration of the esophageal lining can trigger nausea. In some cases, vomiting may be the body's response to alleviate discomfort caused by food impaction.
- **Differentiation:** Persistent vomiting, particularly if bilious or bloody, is more indicative of other conditions such as peptic ulcers, gastric outlet obstruction, or severe infectious processes.

7. Hematemesis (Vomiting Blood) and Melena (Black Stools)

In severe cases of esophagitis, particularly when ulcers are present, bleeding may occur. This can manifest as hematemesis or melena.

- **Mechanism:** Ulcerated or eroded esophageal tissue can bleed, especially when exposed to acidic gastric contents or mechanical trauma from swallowing.
- **Differentiation:** Significant or recurrent bleeding warrants consideration of alternative diagnoses such as peptic ulcer disease, Mallory-Weiss tears, or esophageal varices.

8. Chronic Cough or Sore Throat

Chronic irritation from acid reflux can lead to respiratory or ENT symptoms, including a persistent cough, sore throat, or hoarseness.

- **Mechanism:** Acid reflux into the pharynx or larynx (laryngopharyngeal reflux) causes inflammation and irritation of these structures.
- **Differentiation:** Chronic cough and sore throat related to esophagitis often occur without other respiratory symptoms like fever or nasal congestion, which are common in infections.

9. Weight Loss

Unintentional weight loss may occur in severe or chronic esophagitis, especially when dysphagia or odynophagia limits food intake.

- **Mechanism:** Pain and difficulty swallowing can lead to reduced calorie intake and subsequent weight loss.
- **Differentiation:** Weight loss in esophagitis is gradual and directly related to swallowing difficulties, unlike the more rapid or systemic weight loss seen in malignancies or systemic infections.

Distinguishing Esophagitis from Other GI Disorders

Many gastrointestinal disorders present with overlapping symptoms, making differentiation crucial for accurate diagnosis and treatment. Below are some comparisons:

1. Esophagitis vs. GERD

While GERD is a leading cause of esophagitis, not all GERD cases lead to esophageal inflammation.

- **Key Distinction:** Esophagitis involves visible inflammation of the esophageal lining, confirmed through endoscopy, whereas GERD may only present with reflux symptoms without mucosal damage.

2. Esophagitis vs. Peptic Ulcer Disease

Both conditions can present with epigastric pain and nausea.

- **Key Distinction:** Peptic ulcers cause more localized pain in the upper abdomen, often relieved by food. Esophagitis-related pain is more likely to occur with swallowing and is often retrosternal.

3. Esophagitis vs. Achalasia

Achalasia is a motility disorder that impairs the esophagus's ability to move food toward the stomach.

- **Key Distinction:** Dysphagia in achalasia typically affects both solids and liquids from the onset, while esophagitis-associated dysphagia initially involves solids.

4. Esophagitis vs. Esophageal Cancer

Both conditions can present with progressive dysphagia and weight loss.

- **Key Distinction:** Esophageal cancer is often associated with systemic symptoms such as fatigue and more rapid weight loss. Diagnostic imaging and biopsies are essential for differentiation.

5. Esophagitis vs. Infectious Gastroenteritis

Both may involve nausea, vomiting, and abdominal discomfort.

- **Key Distinction:** Infectious gastroenteritis is usually acute, associated with diarrhea and systemic symptoms like fever, which are not typical in esophagitis.

6. Esophagitis vs. Laryngopharyngeal Reflux (LPR)

LPR involves reflux into the throat and voice box, causing ENT symptoms.

- **Key Distinction:** LPR symptoms such as hoarseness, throat clearing, and postnasal drip predominate over classic esophagitis symptoms like heartburn and dysphagia.

Diagnostic Approaches to Symptom Evaluation

Accurate diagnosis of esophagitis relies on correlating clinical symptoms with diagnostic findings. Key diagnostic tools include:

1. **Endoscopy:** Visual examination of the esophagus to identify inflammation, ulcers, strictures, or other abnormalities.
2. **Biopsy:** Tissue samples taken during endoscopy can confirm eosinophilic esophagitis, infections, or malignancies.
3. **Barium Swallow:** Useful for detecting structural abnormalities like strictures or motility disorders.
4. **pH Monitoring:** Identifies acid reflux and helps differentiate GERD-related esophagitis from other conditions.
5. **Allergy Testing:** Identifies food or environmental triggers in eosinophilic esophagitis.

The symptoms of esophagitis can vary widely in severity and presentation, from mild discomfort to debilitating pain and difficulty swallowing. Recognizing these symptoms and distinguishing them from other GI disorders is vital for effective management. Advanced diagnostic techniques and a thorough clinical history are essential tools in identifying the underlying cause and guiding appropriate treatment.

Chapter 3: How Does Gastroesophageal Reflux Disease (GERD) Contribute to the Development of Esophagitis, and What Are Its Other Underlying Risk Factors?

Gastroesophageal Reflux Disease (GERD) is a prevalent gastrointestinal condition that affects millions of people worldwide. At its core, GERD involves the backward flow of stomach contents into the esophagus, which can lead to significant complications, including esophagitis—the inflammation of the esophageal lining. This chapter explores how GERD contributes to esophagitis, delves into the mechanisms of this interaction, and examines the underlying risk factors that predispose individuals to both conditions.

The Relationship Between GERD and Esophagitis

GERD is the leading cause of esophagitis. The esophagus, a muscular tube connecting the throat to the stomach, is lined with delicate mucosa that is not designed to withstand the acidic and enzymatic contents of the stomach. When reflux occurs, these corrosive contents irritate and damage the esophageal lining, leading to inflammation and, eventually, esophagitis.

1. Mechanism of Acid Reflux-Induced Esophagitis

- **Lower Esophageal Sphincter Dysfunction:** At the junction of the esophagus and stomach lies the lower esophageal sphincter (LES), a circular band of muscle that prevents stomach contents from refluxing into the esophagus. In GERD, the LES becomes weakened or relaxes inappropriately, allowing acid and bile to escape into the esophagus.
- **Erosive Damage:** Repeated exposure to gastric acid, bile salts, and digestive enzymes (such as pepsin) erodes the esophageal lining, resulting in inflammation, pain, and swelling characteristic of esophagitis.
- **Impaired Esophageal Clearance:** The esophagus relies on peristalsis—coordinated

muscular contractions—to move food to the stomach and clear refluxed material. Impaired peristalsis, often observed in GERD, can prolong acid exposure, increasing the risk of esophagitis.
- **Reduced Salivary Defense:** Saliva contains bicarbonate, which helps neutralize acid. GERD patients often have diminished salivary flow or impaired bicarbonate secretion, further exacerbating acid damage.

2. Chronic Exposure and Progression to Complications

Repeated episodes of reflux can lead to chronic esophagitis. Over time, the persistent inflammation can result in complications such as:

- **Esophageal Strictures:** Scarring from repeated injury narrows the esophagus, causing swallowing difficulties (dysphagia).
- **Barrett's Esophagus:** In some individuals, chronic esophagitis leads to cellular changes in the esophageal lining, increasing the risk of esophageal adenocarcinoma.
- **Ulcerations:** Severe inflammation can lead to ulcers, causing bleeding, pain, and additional damage.

Risk Factors for GERD and Esophagitis

Several intrinsic and extrinsic factors contribute to the development of GERD and its progression to esophagitis. Understanding these risk factors is crucial for prevention and management.

1. Lifestyle and Dietary Habits

- **Dietary Triggers:** Certain foods and beverages can weaken the LES or stimulate acid production, increasing reflux risk. Common triggers include:
    - Fatty and fried foods
    - Spicy foods
    - Caffeine and carbonated beverages
    - Alcohol
    - Chocolate
    - Citrus fruits and juices
    - Tomatoes and tomato-based products
- **Meal Patterns:** Eating large meals or lying down shortly after eating can exacerbate reflux. Late-night meals are particularly problematic as they allow gastric contents to linger and reflux during sleep.

2. Obesity

Obesity is a significant risk factor for GERD and esophagitis. Excess body weight increases intra-abdominal pressure, which can:

- Compromise the LES's integrity.
- Promote hiatal hernia formation, a condition that further facilitates acid reflux.
- Prolong acid clearance time by impairing esophageal motility.

3. Hiatal Hernia

A hiatal hernia occurs when the upper part of the stomach pushes through the diaphragm into the chest cavity. This structural abnormality weakens the LES and facilitates reflux, increasing the risk of esophagitis.

- **Types:** Hiatal hernias are classified as sliding (where the stomach and LES move above the diaphragm) or paraesophageal (where part of the stomach bulges alongside the esophagus).
- **Association with GERD:** Sliding hiatal hernias are more commonly associated with GERD and esophagitis due to their direct impact on LES function.

4. Smoking and Alcohol Consumption

Both smoking and alcohol use are independent risk factors for GERD and esophagitis:

- **Smoking:** Nicotine relaxes the LES, reduces saliva production, and impairs esophageal healing, making it a triple threat.

- **Alcohol:** Alcohol irritates the esophageal lining, increases gastric acid secretion, and relaxes the LES, compounding the risk.

5. Medications

Certain medications can increase the likelihood of reflux and esophagitis by relaxing the LES or causing direct mucosal irritation. Common culprits include:

- NSAIDs (e.g., ibuprofen, aspirin)
- Calcium channel blockers (used for hypertension)
- Benzodiazepines (used for anxiety and insomnia)
- Anticholinergics (used for a variety of conditions, including urinary incontinence)
- Bisphosphonates (used for osteoporosis)

6. Pregnancy

Hormonal changes and increased intra-abdominal pressure during pregnancy can lead to transient LES relaxation, making GERD and esophagitis common in pregnant individuals. Symptoms often resolve postpartum.

7. Age-Related Factors

- **Infants and Children:** GERD and esophagitis in this population are often due to developmental immaturity of the LES.

Symptoms include regurgitation, irritability, and feeding difficulties.
- **Older Adults:** Age-related weakening of the LES, decreased esophageal motility, and polypharmacy (use of multiple medications) increase the risk of GERD and esophagitis in elderly populations.

8. Genetic and Familial Factors

Evidence suggests that genetics may play a role in GERD and esophagitis:

- Family history of GERD increases susceptibility.
- Certain genetic conditions, such as connective tissue disorders like scleroderma, predispose individuals to LES dysfunction and reflux.

GERD-Related Complications Leading to Esophagitis

Chronic GERD often sets the stage for severe complications that exacerbate esophagitis. These include:

1. Acid Reflux Severity

Frequent or prolonged episodes of acid reflux increase the likelihood of developing esophagitis. Nighttime reflux is particularly damaging due to:

- Reduced saliva production and swallowing during sleep.
- Prolonged acid contact with the esophageal lining.

2. Bile Reflux

In addition to acid reflux, bile from the duodenum can flow backward into the stomach and esophagus, causing additional irritation and inflammation. Bile reflux is less common but more severe than acid reflux, often leading to significant esophagitis.

3. Delayed Gastric Emptying

Conditions that slow the emptying of stomach contents, such as gastroparesis, increase the risk of reflux and esophagitis. Delayed gastric emptying prolongs the presence of acid in the stomach, enhancing its potential to reflux.

4. Barrett's Esophagus

In some GERD patients, the esophageal lining undergoes metaplasia, transforming into a tissue type more resistant to acid but with a higher risk of malignancy. While this adaptation reduces symptoms, it is often accompanied by chronic esophagitis.

5. Esophageal Motility Disorders

Disorders like achalasia or diffuse esophageal spasm impair peristalsis, leading to prolonged acid exposure and increased risk of esophagitis.

Management and Prevention Strategies

Effectively managing GERD to prevent esophagitis involves a combination of lifestyle changes, medications, and, in severe cases, surgical intervention.

1. Lifestyle Modifications

- Maintain a healthy weight.
- Avoid trigger foods and beverages.
- Eat smaller meals and avoid lying down immediately after eating.
- Elevate the head of the bed to reduce nighttime reflux.
- Quit smoking and limit alcohol consumption.

2. Medications

- **Proton Pump Inhibitors (PPIs):** Reduce gastric acid production and promote esophageal healing.
- **H2 Receptor Antagonists:** Provide symptom relief by lowering stomach acid levels.

- **Antacids:** Offer quick but temporary relief by neutralizing stomach acid.
- **Prokinetics:** Improve gastric emptying and esophageal motility.

3. Surgical Options

For patients with refractory GERD or severe esophagitis, surgical interventions such as fundoplication or LINX device implantation may be considered.

4. Regular Monitoring

Patients with chronic GERD and esophagitis should undergo regular endoscopic evaluations to monitor for complications such as strictures, Barrett's esophagus, or esophageal cancer.

GERD is a primary contributor to the development of esophagitis, with mechanisms rooted in LES dysfunction, acid and bile exposure, and impaired esophageal defenses. A variety of risk factors—ranging from lifestyle habits to structural abnormalities—play a role in exacerbating this condition. Understanding these factors is essential for effective prevention, timely diagnosis, and appropriate management, ultimately reducing the burden of esophagitis and its complications.

Chapter 4: What Are the Differences Between the Various Types of Esophagitis, Such as Eosinophilic Esophagitis, Infectious Esophagitis, and Drug-Induced Esophagitis?

Esophagitis is a condition that encompasses a variety of subtypes, each with distinct causes, clinical features, and treatment approaches. Understanding these differences is crucial for accurate diagnosis and tailored management. This chapter explores the three major types of esophagitis—Eosinophilic Esophagitis (EoE), Infectious Esophagitis, and Drug-Induced Esophagitis—shedding light on their unique characteristics, pathophysiology, and therapeutic strategies.

Eosinophilic Esophagitis (EoE)

Definition and Pathophysiology

Eosinophilic Esophagitis is a chronic, immune-mediated condition characterized by the presence of eosinophils—a type of white blood cell—in the esophageal lining. EoE is primarily driven by allergic reactions to environmental or dietary antigens.

- **Triggers:** Common food allergens, such as dairy, wheat, eggs, soy, and nuts, are frequently implicated. Environmental allergens, like pollen, can also play a role.
- **Mechanism:** Repeated exposure to allergens leads to inflammation and remodeling of the esophageal tissue, resulting in fibrosis and strictures over time.

Clinical Features

- **Symptoms:**
    - Dysphagia (difficulty swallowing), particularly with solid foods.
    - Food impaction (the sensation of food getting stuck in the esophagus).
    - Chest pain or heartburn that mimics GERD but is unresponsive to antacids.
    - In children: Feeding difficulties, vomiting, and failure to thrive.
- **Endoscopic Findings:**

- Rings ("trachealization") in the esophagus.
- Linear furrows.
- White exudates or plaques.
- Narrowing or strictures in advanced cases.

Diagnosis

- **Biopsy:** Histological examination reveals eosinophil infiltration (typically >15 eosinophils per high-power field).
- **Allergy Testing:** Skin prick or blood tests to identify specific food allergens.
- **Exclusion of Other Causes:** Conditions like GERD must be ruled out.

Treatment

- **Dietary Management:**
  - Elimination diets (e.g., six-food elimination diet).
  - Elemental diets, consisting of amino acid-based formulas, are often used for severe cases.
- **Medications:**
  - Topical corticosteroids (e.g., fluticasone or budesonide) to reduce inflammation.
  - Proton pump inhibitors (PPIs) may have anti-inflammatory effects in some patients.

- **Endoscopic Dilation:** Used to treat strictures but does not address underlying inflammation.

Infectious Esophagitis

Definition and Pathophysiology

Infectious Esophagitis occurs when pathogens such as fungi, viruses, or bacteria invade the esophageal lining, leading to inflammation. It is more common in individuals with weakened immune systems, such as those with HIV/AIDS, cancer, or organ transplants.

- **Common Pathogens:**
    - *Candida albicans*: The most frequent cause, especially in immunocompromised individuals.
    - Herpes Simplex Virus (HSV): Causes localized ulcers in the esophagus.
    - Cytomegalovirus (CMV): Often affects individuals with advanced immunosuppression.
    - Rare bacterial infections, often secondary to trauma or other conditions.

Clinical Features

- **Symptoms:**
    - Odynophagia (painful swallowing).

- Dysphagia.
- Retrosternal chest pain.
- Fever and systemic symptoms in severe cases.
- **Endoscopic Findings:**
  - *Candida*: White, adherent plaques resembling "cottage cheese."
  - HSV: Small, vesicular lesions that evolve into ulcers.
  - CMV: Large, shallow ulcers.

Diagnosis

- **Endoscopy with Biopsy:**
  - Provides definitive diagnosis by identifying causative pathogens.
  - Histopathological examination and microbial cultures confirm the etiology.
- **Additional Tests:**
  - Viral PCR testing for HSV and CMV.
  - Blood cultures if systemic infection is suspected.

Treatment

- **Antifungal Therapy:**
  - For *Candida albicans*, first-line treatment includes oral fluconazole or intravenous echinocandins for severe cases.
- **Antiviral Therapy:**

- o HSV: Acyclovir or valacyclovir.
- o CMV: Intravenous ganciclovir, followed by oral valganciclovir.
- **Antibiotics:**
  - o Rarely needed but used for bacterial infections when indicated.

Special Considerations

- Prophylactic antifungal or antiviral therapy may be warranted for immunocompromised individuals at high risk.

Drug-Induced Esophagitis

Definition and Pathophysiology

Drug-Induced Esophagitis occurs when certain medications cause localized damage to the esophageal mucosa. This can result from direct irritation, prolonged contact with the esophageal lining, or systemic effects.

- **Mechanism:**
  - o Pills that dissolve slowly in the esophagus can cause direct irritation.
  - o Medications that lower LES tone or delay gastric emptying can exacerbate reflux and subsequent inflammation.

Common Offending Medications

- Nonsteroidal anti-inflammatory drugs (NSAIDs), such as ibuprofen and aspirin.
- Antibiotics, particularly tetracycline and doxycycline.
- Bisphosphonates, used for osteoporosis (e.g., alendronate).
- Potassium chloride and iron supplements.
- Anticholinergics and calcium channel blockers.

Clinical Features

- **Symptoms:**
    - Sudden-onset chest pain or odynophagia.
    - Dysphagia, often localized to a specific area of the esophagus.
    - Regurgitation of pill fragments in severe cases.
- **Endoscopic Findings:**
    - Ulcers, erosions, or localized inflammation at the site where the pill lodged.

Diagnosis

- **Clinical History:**
    - Strongly suggestive when symptoms occur shortly after starting a new medication.

- Identifying improper pill-taking techniques (e.g., swallowing pills without water or lying down immediately after ingestion).
- **Endoscopy:** Confirms the diagnosis by visualizing the location and extent of damage.

Treatment

- **Immediate Management:**
  - Discontinue the offending medication.
  - Use liquid or alternative formulations if the medication is essential.
- **Symptom Relief:**
  - Proton pump inhibitors (PPIs) or H2 receptor blockers to reduce acid exposure and promote healing.
  - Pain management with topical anesthetics or systemic analgesics.
- **Prevention:**
  - Take pills with a full glass of water.
  - Remain upright for at least 30 minutes after taking medication.

Comparative Analysis of the Three Types

Feature	Eosinophilic Esophagitis	Infectious Esophagitis	Drug-Induced Esophagitis
Primary Cause	Allergic/immune-mediated reaction	Pathogenic infection	Medication-induced mucosal injury
Common Population	Children and young adults	Immunocompromised individuals	Elderly or those with polypharmacy
Key Symptoms	Dysphagia, food impaction	Odynophagia, systemic symptoms	Sudden-onset chest pain, odynophagia
Endoscopic Findings	Rings, furrows, plaques	Plaques (Candida), ulcers (HSV, CMV)	Localized ulcers or erosions
First-Line Treatment	Dietary elimination, corticosteroids	Antifungal/antiviral medications	Discontinuation of offending drug

While all forms of esophagitis share some overlapping symptoms, their underlying causes, clinical features, and management strategies differ significantly. Eosinophilic Esophagitis is primarily driven by allergic reactions and requires a focus on dietary triggers and immune modulation. Infectious Esophagitis, more common in immunocompromised populations, necessitates targeted antimicrobial therapy. Drug-Induced Esophagitis highlights the importance of proper medication administration to prevent injury. Understanding these distinctions enables clinicians to provide effective, patient-specific care and ensures better outcomes for those affected by this diverse condition.

Chapter 5: What Diagnostic Methods Are Used to Confirm Esophagitis, and How Do Endoscopy, Biopsy, and Imaging Techniques Contribute to Accurate Diagnosis?

Accurately diagnosing esophagitis is critical for effective treatment and the prevention of complications. Given the diverse causes and presentations of esophagitis, healthcare providers rely on a combination of clinical evaluation, laboratory tests, endoscopy, biopsies, and imaging techniques to confirm the diagnosis. This chapter delves into the various diagnostic methods used to identify esophagitis, emphasizing how advanced tools such as endoscopy, biopsy, and imaging play a pivotal role in accurate diagnosis and differentiation from other gastrointestinal disorders.

Clinical Evaluation: The First Step

Diagnosis begins with a thorough clinical evaluation, which includes a detailed patient history and physical examination.

Patient History

- **Symptoms Assessment:** Dysphagia (difficulty swallowing), odynophagia (painful swallowing), heartburn, chest pain, regurgitation, and nausea are common symptoms of esophagitis. Recording the duration, severity, and triggers of these symptoms provides crucial clues.
- **Risk Factor Identification:** Healthcare providers inquire about potential risk factors, such as:
    - GERD (gastroesophageal reflux disease).
    - Medication history, including NSAIDs or bisphosphonates.
    - Recent infections or immunosuppressive states.
    - History of allergies or asthma, particularly for eosinophilic esophagitis.
    - Lifestyle habits such as smoking and alcohol consumption.

- **Dietary Triggers:** Identifying food allergies or intolerances may point to eosinophilic esophagitis.

Physical Examination

While physical findings are often nonspecific, clinicians may note:

- Signs of nutritional deficiencies or weight loss.
- Oral thrush, indicative of potential fungal infections like *Candida albicans*.
- Evidence of dehydration or systemic illness in severe cases.

Laboratory Tests

Laboratory investigations provide supportive evidence for the diagnosis of esophagitis.

Blood Tests

- **Eosinophil Count:** Elevated levels may suggest eosinophilic esophagitis.
- **Inflammatory Markers:** High C-reactive protein (CRP) or erythrocyte sedimentation rate (ESR) levels indicate systemic inflammation.
- **Infectious Workup:**
    - HIV testing may be warranted for immunocompromised patients with infectious esophagitis.

o Viral load and antibody testing for HSV or CMV.

Allergy Testing

- **Skin Prick Tests or Serum IgE Levels:** Identify food or environmental allergens in eosinophilic esophagitis.
- **Elimination Diet Trials:** Used to correlate symptom improvement with dietary changes.

Endoscopy: The Gold Standard

Upper endoscopy (esophagogastroduodenoscopy or EGD) is the cornerstone diagnostic tool for esophagitis. It provides direct visualization of the esophageal mucosa, allowing for detailed assessment and targeted biopsy.

Procedure Overview

During endoscopy, a flexible tube with a camera is inserted through the mouth into the esophagus. The procedure is minimally invasive and performed under sedation.

Findings in Esophagitis

Endoscopy reveals characteristic findings for different types of esophagitis:

- **Reflux Esophagitis (GERD):**
  - Erythema (redness) and friability of the esophageal mucosa.
  - Linear erosions and ulcers, typically in the distal esophagus.
  - Complications such as strictures or Barrett's esophagus.
- **Eosinophilic Esophagitis (EoE):**
  - Concentric rings ("trachealization" or "feline esophagus").
  - White exudates or plaques.
  - Linear furrows and narrowing of the esophagus.
- **Infectious Esophagitis:**
  - *Candida albicans:* White, adherent plaques that scrape off easily.
  - HSV: Small, vesicular lesions and "volcano-like" ulcers.
  - CMV: Large, shallow ulcers, often in the mid to distal esophagus.
- **Drug-Induced Esophagitis:**
  - Localized ulcerations or erosions, typically at points of prolonged contact with the offending pill.

Role of Therapeutic Endoscopy

In addition to diagnosis, endoscopy can serve therapeutic purposes, such as dilation of strictures in eosinophilic or chronic reflux esophagitis.

Biopsy: Essential for Histological Confirmation

Histological examination of esophageal tissue obtained during endoscopy is critical for confirming the diagnosis and determining the underlying cause of esophagitis.

Indications for Biopsy

Biopsies are performed to:

- Confirm eosinophilic esophagitis by identifying eosinophil infiltration.
- Distinguish infectious causes (e.g., fungal hyphae, viral inclusion bodies).
- Detect cellular changes associated with Barrett's esophagus or malignancy.

Procedure and Technique

Multiple biopsies are taken from different areas of the esophagus to ensure comprehensive evaluation. Special staining techniques may be used to identify specific pathogens or cellular abnormalities.

Histological Findings

- **Eosinophilic Esophagitis:**
    - 15 eosinophils per high-power field.

- Basal cell hyperplasia and lamina propria fibrosis.
- **Infectious Esophagitis:**
  - *Candida:* Presence of pseudohyphae or yeast forms.
  - HSV: Multinucleated giant cells with inclusion bodies.
  - CMV: Enlarged cells with owl-eye inclusion bodies.
- **Reflux Esophagitis:**
  - Neutrophilic or lymphocytic infiltration.
  - Erosion and ulceration of the mucosa.

Imaging Techniques

Imaging studies complement endoscopy and biopsy in diagnosing esophagitis and identifying complications.

Barium Swallow

Barium swallow is a radiographic study where the patient ingests a barium-containing contrast material, which outlines the esophagus on X-ray.

- **Indications:**
  - Evaluate structural abnormalities, such as strictures or rings.
  - Assess esophageal motility disorders contributing to symptoms.
- **Findings in Esophagitis:**

- Narrowing or strictures in eosinophilic or chronic reflux esophagitis.
- Ulcers or mucosal irregularities.

Computed Tomography (CT)

CT scans are not routinely used for diagnosing esophagitis but are valuable for detecting complications or alternative diagnoses.

- **Indications:**
    - Suspected perforation or abscess.
    - Evaluation of mediastinal structures in severe infections.
- **Findings:**
    - Thickened esophageal wall.
    - Periesophageal inflammation or fluid collections.

Magnetic Resonance Imaging (MRI)

MRI is rarely used but may provide detailed soft tissue imaging in complex cases.

pH Monitoring and Esophageal Manometry

For cases where reflux esophagitis is suspected but not confirmed through endoscopy, additional functional studies may be employed:

- **24-Hour pH Monitoring:** Measures acid exposure in the esophagus over a 24-hour period, helping to confirm GERD as the cause of esophagitis.
- **Esophageal Manometry:** Evaluates esophageal motility and LES pressure, identifying motility disorders that may mimic or exacerbate esophagitis.

Differential Diagnosis

Accurate diagnosis of esophagitis also involves ruling out other conditions with similar presentations, such as:

- Peptic ulcer disease.
- Esophageal cancer.
- Achalasia.
- Functional heartburn or globus sensation.

Diagnosing esophagitis requires a multimodal approach, combining clinical evaluation, laboratory tests, endoscopy, biopsy, and imaging techniques. Endoscopy remains the gold standard, providing direct visualization and allowing for targeted biopsies, while imaging studies and functional tests offer additional insights into structural and functional abnormalities. This comprehensive diagnostic strategy ensures accurate identification of the underlying cause and guides effective management.

Chapter 6: How Is Eosinophilic Esophagitis Diagnosed and Treated, and What Role Do Food Allergies and Elimination Diets Play in Its Management?

Eosinophilic Esophagitis (EoE) is a chronic, immune-mediated inflammatory condition of the esophagus that has emerged as a significant cause of swallowing difficulties and food impaction in both children and adults. This chapter explores the diagnostic processes and treatment options for EoE, with an emphasis on the critical role that food allergies and elimination diets play in managing this condition.

Understanding Eosinophilic Esophagitis

Definition and Epidemiology

EoE is defined as a chronic, antigen-driven inflammatory disease characterized by eosinophil infiltration into the esophageal epithelium. It affects people of all ages but is most commonly diagnosed in children and young adults.

- **Prevalence:**
  - The incidence of EoE has increased over the past two decades, likely due to heightened awareness and improved diagnostic methods.
  - More common in males than females, with a male-to-female ratio of approximately 3:1.
- **Geographic Variation:**
  - EoE is more prevalent in Western countries, possibly due to dietary and environmental differences.

Pathophysiology

EoE is driven by a combination of genetic, environmental, and immune factors. The interaction between food antigens, environmental allergens, and the immune system leads to:

- **Eosinophil Activation:** Elevated levels of eosinophils are recruited to the esophagus in response to antigens, resulting in tissue inflammation and remodeling.
- **Tissue Damage:** Chronic inflammation causes fibrosis, strictures, and impaired esophageal motility, leading to the hallmark symptoms of dysphagia and food impaction.

Diagnosing Eosinophilic Esophagitis

Accurate diagnosis of EoE requires a systematic approach involving clinical evaluation, endoscopy, histopathology, and exclusion of alternative causes of esophageal eosinophilia.

Clinical Presentation

Symptoms in Children

- Feeding difficulties.
- Vomiting.
- Abdominal pain.
- Failure to thrive or weight loss.

Symptoms in Adults

- Dysphagia (difficulty swallowing), particularly with solid foods.
- Food impaction.
- Chest pain mimicking GERD.
- Heartburn and regurgitation resistant to acid suppression therapy.

Diagnostic Criteria

The diagnosis of EoE is established based on the following criteria:

1. Endoscopic Findings

An upper endoscopy (esophagogastroduodenoscopy or EGD) provides direct visualization of the esophagus. Common findings include:

- **Rings:** Concentric, fixed, or transient esophageal rings ("trachealization" or "feline esophagus").
- **Furrows:** Longitudinal furrows or grooves in the mucosa.
- **Exudates:** White plaques or specks that resemble candida infection.
- **Strictures:** Narrowing of the esophageal lumen.
- **Fragility:** Mucosa that tears easily upon biopsy ("crepe paper" appearance).

While these findings are suggestive of EoE, they are not definitive, as some patients may have a normal-appearing esophagus.

2. Histological Examination

Biopsies are the cornerstone of EoE diagnosis. Multiple tissue samples (typically 2-4 from the proximal and distal esophagus) are obtained during endoscopy to ensure adequate assessment.

- **Key Findings:**
    - ≥15 eosinophils per high-power field (HPF) in esophageal tissue.
    - Evidence of basal cell hyperplasia and lamina propria fibrosis.

3. Exclusion of Other Causes

Esophageal eosinophilia can occur in other conditions, such as GERD, infections, connective tissue disorders, and drug reactions. A trial of proton pump inhibitor (PPI) therapy is often used to exclude PPI-responsive esophageal eosinophilia (PPI-REE), a condition that mimics EoE but responds to acid suppression.

Adjunctive Tests

- **Allergy Testing:** Skin prick or serum-specific IgE tests identify potential food and environmental allergens.
- **pH Monitoring:** Evaluates acid exposure to distinguish GERD-related inflammation from EoE.

Treatment of Eosinophilic Esophagitis

The management of EoE aims to alleviate symptoms, reduce inflammation, prevent complications such as strictures, and improve quality of life. Treatment strategies include dietary modifications, pharmacotherapy, and, in some cases, endoscopic interventions.

Dietary Therapy

Dietary management is a cornerstone of EoE treatment, as food antigens are the primary drivers of inflammation.

1. Elimination Diets

Elimination diets identify and remove specific food triggers based on clinical history, allergy testing, or empirical strategies. Common approaches include:

- **Six-Food Elimination Diet (SFED):**
    - Removes the six most common allergens: dairy, wheat, eggs, soy, nuts, and seafood.
    - Patients are monitored for symptom improvement and undergo repeat endoscopy to assess response.
    - Foods are reintroduced sequentially, with endoscopic evaluation to identify triggers.
- **Four-Food or Two-Food Elimination Diets:**
    - Simplified versions of SFED, removing fewer allergens for better patient adherence.
- **Elemental Diet:**
    - Uses amino acid-based formulas to completely eliminate antigen exposure.
    - Highly effective but challenging due to its restrictive nature and cost.

2. Maintenance Diets

Once triggers are identified, a long-term dietary plan is established to prevent recurrence while maintaining nutritional balance.

Pharmacological Therapy

1. Proton Pump Inhibitors (PPIs)

PPIs, such as omeprazole or esomeprazole, are often used as first-line therapy.

- **Mechanism:**
    - Reduce acid exposure, which may contribute to inflammation.
    - Exhibit anti-inflammatory properties independent of acid suppression.
- **Efficacy:** Effective in a subset of patients with PPI-responsive esophageal eosinophilia.

2. Topical Corticosteroids

Topical corticosteroids, delivered through swallowed aerosols or viscous suspensions, directly target esophageal inflammation.

- **Medications:**
    - Fluticasone: Administered as a swallowed inhaler.
    - Budesonide: Mixed with a viscous agent to coat the esophagus.

- **Efficacy:** Reduces eosinophil counts and improves symptoms in most patients.
- **Side Effects:** Minimal systemic absorption; localized effects such as oral candidiasis may occur.

3. Systemic Corticosteroids

Systemic corticosteroids (e.g., prednisone) are reserved for severe, refractory cases due to the risk of significant side effects.

4. Biologic Therapies

Emerging therapies targeting specific immune pathways offer promising alternatives for refractory EoE:

- **Anti-IL-5 Agents:** Reduce eosinophil recruitment (e.g., mepolizumab, reslizumab).
- **Anti-IL-13/IL-4 Agents:** Target cytokines involved in inflammation (e.g., dupilumab).

Endoscopic Management

1. Dilation

Esophageal dilation is used to treat strictures or narrow-caliber esophagus, improving swallowing.

- **Procedure:** Involves mechanical stretching of the esophagus under sedation.

- **Risks:** Rare complications include perforation or bleeding.
- **Limitations:** Does not address underlying inflammation.

Monitoring and Long-Term Management

EoE is a chronic condition requiring regular monitoring to prevent complications.

- **Follow-Up Endoscopy:** Assess treatment response and monitor for disease progression.
- **Symptom Monitoring:** Patients are encouraged to report any recurrence of symptoms promptly.

The Role of Food Allergies and Elimination Diets

Importance of Food Allergies

Food allergens play a central role in the pathogenesis of EoE. Identifying and eliminating specific triggers can:

- Reduce inflammation and eosinophil infiltration.
- Improve symptoms and prevent disease progression.

Challenges in Implementing Elimination Diets

- **Adherence:** Strict dietary restrictions can be difficult to maintain.
- **Nutritional Deficiencies:** Elimination of multiple food groups may require dietary supplements or nutritionist support.
- **Repeat Endoscopy:** Necessary to confirm the effectiveness of dietary changes, adding cost and inconvenience.

Advances in Diet-Based Management

- **Personalized Diets:** Advances in allergy testing and dietary response evaluation enable tailored elimination strategies.
- **Non-Invasive Monitoring:** Biomarkers and minimally invasive tests (e.g., esophageal string test) are being developed to reduce the need for repeat endoscopy.

Eosinophilic Esophagitis is a complex condition requiring a multidisciplinary approach to diagnosis and treatment. Accurate identification of food triggers and the implementation of elimination diets are central to effective management. Advances in pharmacological therapies and endoscopic techniques provide additional options for refractory cases. With continued research and innovation, the management of EoE is evolving toward more personalized, patient-centered care.

Chapter 7: The Esophagitis Solution: Strategies for Recovery and Prevention

Esophagitis, the inflammation of the esophagus, can significantly impact quality of life if left untreated. From painful swallowing to long-term complications like strictures or Barrett's esophagus, managing and preventing this condition requires a multi-faceted approach. This chapter explores actionable strategies for treating esophagitis and preventing its recurrence, emphasizing lifestyle modifications, dietary interventions, medical treatments, and alternative therapies.

Understanding Esophagitis and Its Triggers

To effectively address esophagitis, it is essential to understand its root causes and triggers. The condition commonly arises due to:

- **Gastroesophageal Reflux Disease (GERD):** Chronic acid reflux is the leading cause of esophagitis.

- **Eosinophilic Esophagitis (EoE):** An immune-mediated condition often triggered by food allergens.
- **Infectious Esophagitis:** Caused by fungal, viral, or bacterial infections, particularly in immunocompromised individuals.
- **Drug-Induced Esophagitis:** Resulting from medications that irritate the esophageal lining or remain lodged in the esophagus.
- **Chemical or Physical Injuries:** From accidental ingestion of caustic substances or physical trauma.

By addressing these underlying causes, effective recovery and prevention strategies can be implemented.

Strategies for Recovery

1. Lifestyle Modifications

Lifestyle changes are foundational for managing esophagitis and preventing further irritation of the esophageal lining.

A. Weight Management

- **Why It Matters:** Obesity increases intra-abdominal pressure, worsening acid reflux and GERD-related esophagitis.
- **Action Plan:**
    - Adopt a calorie-controlled diet.

- Engage in regular physical activity, aiming for at least 150 minutes of moderate exercise per week.
- Avoid crash diets or extreme weight loss methods, which can exacerbate GERD symptoms.

B. Posture and Sleep Habits

- **Why It Matters:** Certain positions exacerbate acid reflux.
- **Action Plan:**
  - Avoid lying down within two to three hours after eating.
  - Elevate the head of your bed by 6-8 inches to reduce nighttime reflux.
  - Sleep on your left side to minimize acid exposure in the esophagus.

C. Smoking and Alcohol Cessation

- **Why It Matters:** Smoking relaxes the lower esophageal sphincter (LES), while alcohol increases acid production and irritates the esophageal lining.
- **Action Plan:**
  - Seek smoking cessation programs or nicotine replacement therapies.
  - Limit alcohol consumption to moderate levels or eliminate it entirely.

2. Dietary Interventions

Diet plays a critical role in both the recovery and prevention of esophagitis. Specific dietary adjustments can alleviate symptoms and reduce inflammation.

A. Identifying Trigger Foods

- **Common Triggers:**
    - Acidic foods: Citrus fruits, tomatoes.
    - Spicy foods: Peppers, chili-based dishes.
    - Fatty foods: Fried foods, high-fat dairy.
    - Beverages: Coffee, carbonated drinks, alcohol.
- **Action Plan:**
    - Maintain a food diary to track symptom flare-ups and identify triggers.
    - Eliminate or minimize identified triggers.

B. Adopting an Anti-Inflammatory Diet

- **Why It Matters:** Reduces esophageal inflammation and promotes healing.
- **Action Plan:**
    - Increase intake of fruits and vegetables (non-acidic options like bananas and spinach).
    - Incorporate omega-3 fatty acids from fish, walnuts, or flaxseeds.

- Avoid processed foods and added sugars.

C. Modifying Eating Habits

- **Why It Matters:** Large meals and improper eating habits worsen reflux.
- **Action Plan:**
  - Eat smaller, more frequent meals.
  - Chew food thoroughly to ease swallowing.
  - Avoid eating late at night.

3. Medical Treatments

For moderate to severe cases of esophagitis, medical intervention is often necessary.

A. Proton Pump Inhibitors (PPIs)

- **Why They're Effective:** Reduce stomach acid production, allowing the esophagus to heal.
- **Examples:** Omeprazole, esomeprazole, lansoprazole.
- **Usage:** Follow prescribed dosages and treatment durations, as long-term use may have side effects such as bone loss or nutrient deficiencies.

B. H2 Receptor Antagonists

- **Why They're Effective:** Block histamine receptors in the stomach lining, reducing acid production.
- **Examples:** Ranitidine (withdrawn in some countries), famotidine.
- **Usage:** Suitable for mild to moderate symptoms.

C. Topical or Systemic Corticosteroids

- **Indication:** Used for eosinophilic esophagitis to reduce immune-mediated inflammation.
- **Examples:** Fluticasone (swallowed inhaler), budesonide (viscous suspension).
- **Precaution:** Monitor for side effects like oral thrush.

D. Antifungal, Antiviral, or Antibiotic Therapy

- **Indication:** For infectious esophagitis caused by pathogens like *Candida albicans*, HSV, or CMV.
- **Action Plan:** Tailored treatment based on the identified organism.

E. Prokinetic Agents

- **Why They're Effective:** Improve esophageal motility and gastric emptying, reducing reflux episodes.
- **Examples:** Metoclopramide, domperidone (availability varies).

4. Endoscopic and Surgical Interventions

In cases where medical treatment fails or complications arise, procedural interventions may be necessary.

A. Esophageal Dilation

- **Indication:** For strictures or narrowing caused by chronic inflammation or fibrosis.
- **Procedure:** Mechanical or balloon dilation under endoscopic guidance.
- **Risk:** Small chance of perforation; should be performed by experienced professionals.

B. Fundoplication Surgery

- **Indication:** For refractory GERD leading to esophagitis.
- **Procedure:** Reinforces the LES by wrapping the upper stomach around it.
- **Outcome:** Reduces reflux and prevents esophagitis recurrence.

Strategies for Prevention

1. Maintaining Long-Term Dietary and Lifestyle Changes

Sustained adherence to dietary and lifestyle modifications is crucial to preventing esophagitis recurrence. Patients should:

- Continue avoiding identified trigger foods.
- Practice mindful eating habits.
- Maintain a healthy weight and active lifestyle.

2. Periodic Medical Monitoring

Regular follow-ups with a healthcare provider can identify early signs of recurrence or complications, ensuring timely intervention.

A. Endoscopic Surveillance

- **Indication:** For patients with a history of severe esophagitis, strictures, or Barrett's esophagus.
- **Frequency:** Determined based on individual risk factors.

B. Symptom Tracking

- **Action Plan:** Report new or worsening symptoms, such as difficulty swallowing, persistent heartburn, or unexplained weight loss.

3. Medication Management

- Use medications like PPIs or H2 blockers as prescribed.
- Avoid unnecessary use of NSAIDs and other irritant medications.

- Follow proper pill-swallowing techniques (e.g., take pills with water and remain upright for at least 30 minutes).

4. Preventing Infectious Esophagitis

For immunocompromised individuals:

- Maintain good oral hygiene to reduce fungal overgrowth.
- Use prophylactic antiviral or antifungal medications as recommended.
- Manage underlying conditions, such as HIV, to improve immune function.

Alternative and Complementary Therapies

While conventional treatments form the backbone of esophagitis management, some patients may benefit from complementary approaches:

1. Herbal Remedies

- **Slippery Elm:** Forms a protective coating in the esophagus.
- **Chamomile Tea:** May reduce inflammation and promote relaxation.

2. Mind-Body Interventions

- **Stress Management:** Stress can exacerbate GERD and other triggers of esophagitis.
- **Techniques:** Practice yoga, meditation, or deep breathing exercises.

3. Probiotics

- May support gut health and reduce inflammation, particularly for infectious or antibiotic-associated esophagitis.

Recovering from esophagitis and preventing its recurrence requires a comprehensive, individualized approach. By addressing lifestyle factors, dietary triggers, and underlying medical conditions, patients can achieve lasting relief and reduce their risk of complications. Regular follow-ups, adherence to prescribed treatments, and proactive prevention strategies are essential to maintaining esophageal health.

Chapter 8: What Are the Key Treatment Options for Esophagitis, Including Lifestyle Modifications, Medications, and, in Severe Cases, Surgical Interventions?

Esophagitis is a condition that can range from mild discomfort to severe complications affecting swallowing and overall quality of life. The treatment of esophagitis requires a comprehensive approach tailored to the underlying cause, severity, and patient-specific factors. This chapter explores the key treatment options, including lifestyle modifications, medications, and surgical interventions, offering a complete guide for effective management.

Understanding Esophagitis

Esophagitis refers to inflammation of the esophagus and can arise from several causes:

- **Gastroesophageal Reflux Disease (GERD):** The most common cause, involving the backward flow of stomach acid into the esophagus.
- **Eosinophilic Esophagitis (EoE):** An immune-mediated condition often triggered by allergens.
- **Infectious Esophagitis:** Resulting from fungal, viral, or bacterial infections, especially in immunocompromised individuals.
- **Drug-Induced Esophagitis:** Caused by certain medications that irritate the esophagus or get lodged during swallowing.
- **Chemical or Physical Injuries:** From ingestion of caustic substances or physical trauma.

Effective treatment aims to address the root cause, alleviate symptoms, promote healing, and prevent complications like strictures or Barrett's esophagus.

Lifestyle Modifications

Lifestyle changes are the foundation of esophagitis treatment and can significantly reduce symptoms and promote healing.

1. Dietary Adjustments

A. Identifying and Avoiding Trigger Foods

- **Common Triggers:** Spicy foods, acidic foods (citrus, tomatoes), caffeine, carbonated beverages, alcohol, and high-fat meals.
- **Action Plan:** Maintain a food diary to identify individual triggers and eliminate them from the diet.

B. Adopting an Anti-Inflammatory Diet

- Increase intake of anti-inflammatory foods such as leafy greens, nuts, and omega-3-rich fish.
- Limit processed foods and added sugars.

C. Smaller, Frequent Meals

- Avoid large meals that increase intra-abdominal pressure and exacerbate reflux.
- Eat smaller, more frequent meals to minimize esophageal irritation.

2. Postural and Behavioral Modifications

A. Post-Meal Practices

- Avoid lying down within 2-3 hours after eating to reduce acid reflux.

- Elevate the head of the bed by 6-8 inches to minimize nighttime reflux.

B. Smoking and Alcohol

- Quit smoking to improve LES (lower esophageal sphincter) function and reduce esophageal irritation.
- Limit or avoid alcohol, which can relax the LES and irritate the mucosa.

3. Weight Management

A. Obesity and Esophagitis

- Excess abdominal fat increases intra-abdominal pressure, worsening reflux.

B. Action Plan

- Adopt a calorie-controlled diet.
- Engage in regular physical activity (at least 150 minutes of moderate exercise per week).

4. Proper Medication Use

A. Avoiding Pill-Induced Esophagitis

- Swallow pills with a full glass of water.
- Avoid lying down immediately after taking medication.

Medications

Medications play a pivotal role in treating esophagitis by addressing inflammation, reducing acid exposure, and managing symptoms. The choice of medication depends on the underlying cause of esophagitis.

1. Proton Pump Inhibitors (PPIs)

A. Mechanism of Action

- PPIs block the hydrogen-potassium ATPase enzyme in stomach lining cells, reducing gastric acid production.

B. Indications

- GERD-related esophagitis.
- Adjunct therapy in eosinophilic esophagitis.

C. Common PPIs

- Omeprazole, esomeprazole, lansoprazole, pantoprazole.

D. Usage

- Take PPIs before meals for maximum effectiveness.
- Long-term use requires monitoring for potential side effects like bone density loss and vitamin B12 deficiency.

2. H2 Receptor Antagonists

A. Mechanism of Action

- Block histamine receptors in the stomach, reducing acid production.

B. Indications

- Mild to moderate GERD symptoms.

C. Examples

- Ranitidine (withdrawn in some countries), famotidine, cimetidine.

3. Topical Corticosteroids

A. Indications

- Eosinophilic esophagitis to reduce inflammation caused by eosinophil infiltration.

B. Medications

- Fluticasone (swallowed inhaler), budesonide (viscous solution).

C. Administration

- Ensure proper swallowing technique to coat the esophagus.

D. Side Effects

- Localized effects like oral thrush; systemic absorption is minimal.

4. Antifungal, Antiviral, or Antibiotic Therapy

A. Indications

- Infectious esophagitis caused by pathogens like *Candida albicans* (fungal), HSV (viral), or bacterial infections.

B. Medications

- **Fungal:** Fluconazole, itraconazole.
- **Viral:** Acyclovir, ganciclovir.
- **Bacterial:** Antibiotics tailored to the causative organism.

5. Antacids

A. Mechanism of Action

- Neutralize stomach acid, providing quick relief for mild symptoms.

B. Usage

- Over-the-counter antacids like calcium carbonate or magnesium hydroxide are suitable for occasional use.

6. Prokinetic Agents

A. Mechanism of Action

- Improve esophageal motility and gastric emptying, reducing reflux.

B. Examples

- Metoclopramide, domperidone (availability varies).

Surgical Interventions

For severe or refractory esophagitis, surgical options may be necessary. Surgery is typically reserved for patients who fail to respond to medical therapy or have complications such as strictures or Barrett's esophagus.

1. Fundoplication

A. Indication

- Refractory GERD causing chronic esophagitis.

B. Procedure

- The upper part of the stomach is wrapped around the LES to strengthen it and prevent reflux.

C. Types

- Nissen Fundoplication (360-degree wrap).
- Partial Fundoplication (e.g., Toupet, Dor).

D. Outcome

- High success rates in reducing reflux and esophagitis recurrence.

2. Esophageal Dilation

A. Indication

- Esophageal strictures resulting from chronic inflammation or fibrosis.

B. Procedure

- Endoscopic dilation uses balloons or mechanical dilators to stretch the esophagus.

C. Risks

- Perforation and bleeding, though rare.

3. LINX Reflux Management System

A. Indication

- Alternative to fundoplication for GERD-related esophagitis.

B. Procedure

- Magnetic beads are placed around the LES to improve its function while allowing food passage.

4. Esophagectomy

A. Indication

- Rarely required, reserved for severe cases of refractory esophagitis or malignancy.

B. Procedure

- Surgical removal of the damaged esophagus and reconstruction using stomach or intestinal tissue.

Alternative and Complementary Therapies

While conventional treatments form the backbone of esophagitis management, some patients may benefit from complementary approaches.

1. Herbal Remedies

- **Slippery Elm:** Coats and soothes the esophageal lining.
- **Marshmallow Root:** Reduces inflammation.

2. Stress Management

- **Why It Matters:** Stress exacerbates GERD and EoE symptoms.
- **Techniques:** Meditation, yoga, and deep breathing exercises.

3. Probiotics

- **Potential Benefit:** May help in managing infectious or antibiotic-associated esophagitis by improving gut health.

Monitoring and Long-Term Management

Managing esophagitis is an ongoing process, especially for chronic or recurrent cases.

1. Regular Follow-Ups

- Monitor symptoms and treatment efficacy.
- Adjust medications or lifestyle modifications as needed.

2. Endoscopic Surveillance

- Recommended for patients with a history of severe esophagitis or Barrett's esophagus.
- Frequency depends on individual risk factors.

3. Patient Education

- Teach patients about trigger factors, medication adherence, and recognizing warning signs of complications.

Effective treatment of esophagitis requires a holistic approach that combines lifestyle changes, pharmacological therapies, and, in severe cases, surgical interventions. By addressing the underlying causes and empowering patients with knowledge and actionable strategies, the recurrence of esophagitis can be minimized, ensuring long-term esophageal health.

Chapter 9: How Can Esophagitis Be Prevented, and What Steps Can Individuals Take to Minimize Their Risk of Developing This Condition?

Esophagitis, characterized by inflammation of the esophageal lining, can be a debilitating condition if not addressed early. While treatment options are effective in managing the condition, prevention is always preferable. Preventative strategies focus on reducing exposure to known risk factors, maintaining a healthy lifestyle, and addressing underlying medical conditions. This chapter explores the actionable steps individuals can take to minimize their risk of developing esophagitis and its associated complications.

Understanding Esophagitis and Its Risk Factors

Prevention begins with a clear understanding of the causes and risk factors for esophagitis. The major types of esophagitis and their associated triggers include:

1. **Reflux Esophagitis:** Resulting from gastroesophageal reflux disease (GERD), caused by stomach acid repeatedly damaging the esophagus.
2. **Eosinophilic Esophagitis (EoE):** An allergic condition triggered by certain foods or environmental allergens.
3. **Infectious Esophagitis:** Occurring primarily in immunocompromised individuals, caused by fungal, viral, or bacterial infections.
4. **Drug-Induced Esophagitis:** Caused by medications that irritate the esophagus or become lodged during swallowing.
5. **Chemical or Physical Injury:** Resulting from the ingestion of caustic substances or physical trauma to the esophagus.

By addressing these underlying causes and their associated risk factors, esophagitis can often be prevented or its severity significantly reduced

Lifestyle Modifications for Prevention

Lifestyle changes are among the most effective ways to prevent esophagitis. These changes focus on reducing risk factors like acid reflux, exposure to allergens, and poor dietary habits.

1. Dietary Adjustments

A. Avoid Trigger Foods

Certain foods can irritate the esophagus or exacerbate acid reflux, increasing the risk of esophagitis.

- **Common Triggers:**
    - Acidic foods (e.g., citrus fruits, tomatoes).
    - Spicy foods.
    - High-fat or fried foods.
    - Carbonated beverages.
    - Caffeinated drinks (e.g., coffee, tea).
    - Alcohol and chocolate.
- **Action Plan:** Maintain a food diary to identify and eliminate individual triggers.

B. Adopt Healthy Eating Habits

- **Small, Frequent Meals:** Reduces the risk of overeating and minimizes pressure on the lower esophageal sphincter (LES).
- **Chew Thoroughly:** Eases the swallowing process and prevents irritation.
- **Avoid Eating Before Bedtime:** Stop eating 2-3 hours before lying down to reduce nighttime acid reflux.

C. Anti-Inflammatory Diet

Incorporate foods that promote healing and reduce inflammation:

- Leafy greens, broccoli, and non-citrus fruits.
- Omega-3 fatty acids from fish, flaxseeds, or walnuts.
- Whole grains and fiber-rich foods to aid digestion.

2. Weight Management

A. Importance of Healthy Weight

Excess body weight, particularly around the abdomen, increases intra-abdominal pressure, pushing stomach contents into the esophagus.

B. Action Plan

- **Calorie-Controlled Diet:** Focus on nutrient-dense foods.
- **Regular Exercise:** Aim for at least 150 minutes of moderate activity per week.
- **Monitor Progress:** Use tools like BMI calculators and waist measurements to track changes.

3. Smoking and Alcohol Cessation

A. Effects on the Esophagus

- Smoking weakens the LES, allowing stomach acid to reflux into the esophagus.

- Alcohol irritates the esophageal lining and increases acid production.

B. Steps to Quit

- Enroll in smoking cessation programs.
- Use nicotine replacement therapies or prescription medications as needed.
- Limit alcohol intake or avoid it altogether.

4. Posture and Physical Habits

A. Avoid Lying Down After Meals

- **Why It Helps:** Reduces the likelihood of acid reflux by keeping stomach contents in place.
- **Action Plan:** Stay upright for at least 2-3 hours after eating.

B. Sleep Position

- **Elevate the Head of the Bed:** Use blocks or a wedge pillow to raise the head by 6-8 inches, reducing nighttime reflux.
- **Sleep on the Left Side:** This position minimizes acid exposure to the esophagus.

5. Proper Pill-Swallowing Techniques

A. Risk of Drug-Induced Esophagitis

Certain medications can irritate the esophagus or become lodged, causing localized damage.

B. Best Practices

- Swallow pills with a full glass of water.
- Avoid lying down immediately after taking medication.
- Ask for liquid or dissolvable formulations if swallowing pills is difficult.

Addressing Medical Conditions

Managing underlying medical conditions is essential for preventing esophagitis, especially when these conditions increase susceptibility to the disease.

1. Gastroesophageal Reflux Disease (GERD)

A. Importance of GERD Management

Chronic acid reflux damages the esophageal lining, leading to reflux esophagitis.

B. Action Plan

- Use medications like proton pump inhibitors (PPIs) or H2 receptor antagonists as prescribed.

- Follow GERD-specific lifestyle changes, such as avoiding trigger foods and eating smaller meals.

2. Allergies and Eosinophilic Esophagitis (EoE)

A. Role of Allergies

Food allergens are a significant trigger for EoE.

B. Elimination Diets

- **Six-Food Elimination Diet (SFED):** Removes dairy, wheat, eggs, soy, nuts, and seafood.
- **Elemental Diet:** Uses amino acid-based formulas for severe cases.
- **Allergy Testing:** Helps identify specific triggers for personalized dietary modifications.

3. Immunocompromised States

A. Risk of Infectious Esophagitis

Individuals with weakened immune systems (e.g., due to HIV, cancer, or organ transplantation) are at higher risk of infections.

B. Prevention Strategies

- Maintain good oral hygiene to prevent fungal infections.
- Use prophylactic antifungal or antiviral medications when recommended.
- Address underlying immune deficiencies with appropriate treatments.

4. Managing Medications

A. Medications That Irritate the Esophagus

- NSAIDs, bisphosphonates, potassium chloride, and iron supplements are common culprits.

B. Prevention Tips

- Take medications with food if permitted.
- Use enteric-coated formulations to reduce irritation.

Environmental and Behavioral Factors

1. Avoiding Exposure to Caustic Substances

A. Household Safety

- Store cleaning agents and chemicals out of reach of children.

- Use clearly labeled containers to prevent accidental ingestion.

B. Workplace Precautions

- Follow safety protocols when handling hazardous substances.
- Wear protective equipment as needed.

2. Stress Management

A. Link Between Stress and Esophagitis

Stress can exacerbate GERD symptoms and trigger EoE flares.

B. Stress-Reduction Techniques

- Practice mindfulness or meditation.
- Engage in hobbies or physical activities to unwind.
- Seek professional counseling if needed.

Long-Term Prevention and Monitoring

1. Regular Medical Check-Ups

- Schedule periodic visits with a healthcare provider to monitor symptoms and treatment efficacy.

- Undergo endoscopy if symptoms worsen or if you are at risk for complications like Barrett's esophagus.

2. Symptom Awareness

- Recognize early signs of esophagitis, such as difficulty swallowing or persistent heartburn, and seek medical advice promptly.

3. Patient Education

- Understand the importance of adherence to lifestyle modifications and medication regimens.
- Stay informed about new treatments and preventive measures.

Preventing esophagitis involves a proactive approach to minimizing risk factors, managing underlying conditions, and adopting a healthy lifestyle. By implementing these strategies, individuals can significantly reduce their risk of developing esophagitis and improve their overall esophageal health. Regular medical monitoring and a commitment to preventative care are key to achieving long-term well-being.

Chapter 10: Esophagitis: A Comprehensive Clinical Guide for Patients and Practitioners

Esophagitis, a condition characterized by inflammation of the esophagus, can significantly impact the quality of life, causing symptoms that range from mild discomfort to severe pain and difficulty swallowing. This comprehensive guide is designed for both medical professionals and patients, providing detailed information on the causes, symptoms, diagnostic methods, treatment options, and preventive strategies for esophagitis. By bridging clinical insights with patient-centric advice, this chapter aims to empower readers with the knowledge to manage and prevent this condition effectively.

Understanding Esophagitis

Definition

Esophagitis refers to inflammation of the esophageal lining, which may result from various causes, including acid reflux, allergic reactions, infections, and medication-induced injuries. The condition can lead to complications such as ulcers, strictures, and, in chronic cases, Barrett's esophagus, which increases the risk of esophageal cancer.

Types of Esophagitis

1. **Reflux Esophagitis:** Caused by chronic acid reflux (GERD).
2. **Eosinophilic Esophagitis (EoE):** An immune-mediated condition triggered by allergens.
3. **Infectious Esophagitis:** Resulting from infections such as *Candida albicans*, HSV, or CMV, typically in immunocompromised individuals.
4. **Drug-Induced Esophagitis:** Caused by medications that irritate the esophageal lining.
5. **Chemical or Physical Injury:** From ingestion of caustic substances or physical trauma.

Causes and Risk Factors

Common Causes

- **Gastroesophageal Reflux Disease (GERD):** Chronic exposure to stomach acid damages the esophageal lining.
- **Food Allergies:** A major factor in EoE, with triggers like dairy, wheat, and soy.

- **Infections:** Common in individuals with weakened immune systems.
- **Medications:** Pills such as NSAIDs, bisphosphonates, and antibiotics can irritate the esophagus.
- **Chemical Ingestion:** Accidental or intentional ingestion of harmful substances.

Risk Factors

- Obesity.
- Smoking and alcohol use.
- Poor dietary habits, including high-fat or spicy foods.
- Immune suppression (e.g., due to HIV, cancer, or organ transplantation).
- Genetic predisposition, particularly in EoE.

Symptoms of Esophagitis

Common Symptoms

- Dysphagia (difficulty swallowing).
- Odynophagia (painful swallowing).
- Heartburn and chest pain.
- Regurgitation of food or sour liquid.
- Nausea and vomiting.

Severe Symptoms

- Food impaction (food stuck in the esophagus).

- Bleeding (hematemesis or melena).
- Weight loss due to feeding difficulties.

Differentiating Symptoms by Type

- **Reflux Esophagitis:** Predominantly heartburn and regurgitation.
- **EoE:** Dysphagia and food impaction, often in younger patients.
- **Infectious Esophagitis:** Severe odynophagia with systemic symptoms like fever.
- **Drug-Induced Esophagitis:** Sudden-onset chest pain after taking medication.

Diagnostic Methods

1. Clinical Evaluation

- Detailed patient history to identify symptoms, risk factors, and potential triggers.
- Physical examination to assess general health and identify related conditions.

2. Endoscopy

- **Purpose:** Direct visualization of the esophageal lining.
- **Findings:**
    - Erythema, erosions, or ulcers in reflux esophagitis.

- o Rings, furrows, and plaques in EoE.
- o White plaques or shallow ulcers in infectious esophagitis.
- **Biopsy:** Tissue samples confirm diagnosis and rule out malignancy.

3. Laboratory Tests

- **Eosinophil Count:** Elevated levels suggest EoE.
- **Infectious Workup:** Cultures and PCR for fungal, viral, or bacterial pathogens.
- **Allergy Testing:** Identifies triggers in EoE.

4. Imaging

- **Barium Swallow:** Detects structural abnormalities like strictures or rings.
- **CT or MRI:** Evaluates complications such as perforations or abscesses.

5. Functional Tests

- **24-Hour pH Monitoring:** Confirms GERD-related esophagitis.
- **Esophageal Manometry:** Assesses motility disorders contributing to symptoms.

Treatment Options

Lifestyle Modifications

- **Dietary Adjustments:** Avoid trigger foods; adopt smaller, frequent meals.
- **Posture and Habits:** Avoid lying down after meals; elevate the head of the bed.
- **Smoking and Alcohol:** Cessation reduces esophageal irritation.

Medications

1. Proton Pump Inhibitors (PPIs)

- First-line treatment for reflux esophagitis.
- Examples: Omeprazole, esomeprazole.
- Reduces acid production, allowing healing of the esophageal lining.

2. H2 Receptor Antagonists

- Suitable for mild GERD symptoms.
- Examples: Famotidine, ranitidine (withdrawn in some regions).

3. Corticosteroids

- Topical agents like fluticasone or budesonide for EoE.
- Systemic steroids for severe cases.

4. Antifungal, Antiviral, or Antibiotic Therapy

- Tailored to treat infectious esophagitis based on the causative pathogen.

5. Prokinetic Agents

- Improves esophageal motility in patients with motility disorders.

Endoscopic and Surgical Interventions

- **Esophageal Dilation:** For strictures caused by chronic inflammation.
- **Fundoplication:** Surgical reinforcement of the LES for refractory GERD.
- **LINX Reflux Management System:** Magnetic device to improve LES function.

Preventive Strategies

Dietary and Lifestyle Changes

- Avoid trigger foods and large meals.
- Maintain a healthy weight.
- Quit smoking and limit alcohol consumption.

Proper Medication Use

- Swallow pills with water and remain upright afterward.
- Use liquid formulations if swallowing is difficult.

Medical Monitoring

- Regular check-ups for patients with chronic conditions like GERD or EoE.
- Endoscopic surveillance for high-risk patients (e.g., Barrett's esophagus).

Managing Underlying Conditions

- Treat allergies to prevent EoE.
- Address immune suppression to reduce infection risk.

Patient Education and Support

Understanding the Condition

- Patients should be informed about the causes, symptoms, and potential complications of esophagitis.

Adherence to Treatment Plans

- Emphasize the importance of lifestyle changes and medication compliance.
- Educate on recognizing early warning signs of complications.

Access to Resources

- Provide dietary guides, support groups, and counseling services.

Esophagitis is a multifaceted condition requiring a collaborative approach between patients and practitioners. By combining clinical expertise with patient empowerment, effective management and prevention are achievable. This comprehensive guide serves as a roadmap for navigating the complexities of esophagitis, ensuring optimal outcomes for all stakeholders.

Thank You for Reading

Dear Reader,
Thank you for reading the book. If you enjoyed this book or found it useful, I'd be very grateful if you'd post a short review. Your support really does make a difference, and I read all the reviews personally so I can get your feedback and make this book even better. If this book resonated with you or inspired new perspectives, please consider supporting future projects and publications. Your generous contributions make it possible to continue creating meaningful content.

Support My Work:

Venmo: @Nileshlp
Cash App: $drnileshlp

BTC

bc1qs72228z6pauw3rk9tej9f6umu4y9gz289y3cvn

ETH

0xE1DAE6F656c900a4b24257b587ac0856E1e346D2

Every bit of support goes a long way in sustaining my passion for storytelling and public health advocacy. Once again, thank you from the bottom of my heart. Your encouragement and generosity mean the world to me.

Warm regards,
Dr. Nilesh Panchal
Author and Public Health Practitioner

Printed in Great Britain
by Amazon